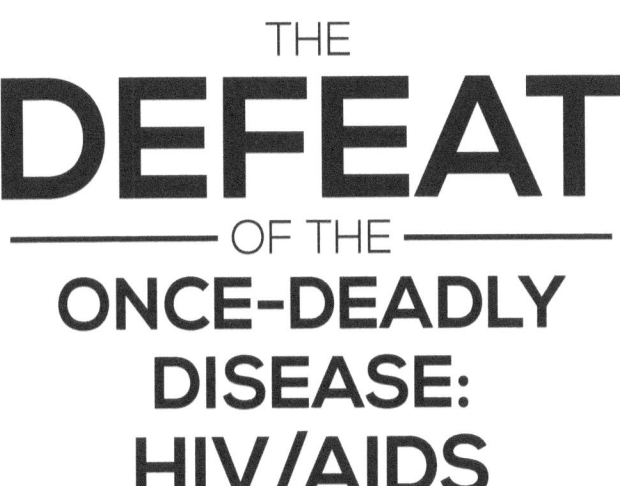

THE

DEFEAT

— OF THE —

ONCE-DEADLY
DISEASE:
HIV/AIDS

THE DEFEAT

OF THE

ONCE-DEADLY DISEASE: HIV/AIDS

CATHERINE ELEBO

To order additional copies of this book, contact:
Xlibris LLC
1-888-795-4274
www.Xlibris.com
Orders@Xlibris.com
136863

Dedication

This book is dedicated to my late husband Edwin Elebo, and to all my children, pastor Edwin-Great, Kingsley, Alex, Ada, and Kennedy. Most importantly to my grand children, Treasure, Victor, Precious, and Prince, for all their unfailing love, encouragement and support they always give me.

Chapter One

After many years of the then unknown virus, many leading scientists during its thirtieth anniversary, could now say that the end of the pandemic is possible. Compared to the early 1980s during the outbreak of the disease that killed many people, we could gladly say that the defeat of the HIV/AIDS epidemic had been achieved as it is no more a death threat. Possibly in a short period, we should be saying "Rest in Peace (R.I.P) HIV" (Hofmann 2011).

There are still at present many people in the world who are HIV positive but are on hiding and many not aware of their HIV status because they are afraid to be tested because of the stigma and ignorance attached to the disease. But as we move from one nation to another and interact with one another with the disease, it continues to go round the whole world, causing damages, for HIV is not written on anyone's face.

The disease does not know your race, ethnicity, gender, sexual orientation, or socioeconomic status, and as we continue to interact in the real world without sexual protection, so does HIV move with us. That is why there has been a crusade to fight HIV/AIDS to finish by getting everyone to be tested from time to time.

Everyone has to be careful on his/her sexual communication for though sex is part of life, we cannot stop human beings from sexuality; rather, we have to be wise with our sexual partners. The greatest achievement for us in this life is to love oneself: if you love yourself, it is important to get tested today for HIV. The disease is everywhere in the whole world, and to be free of it, you are to be aware of it, fight it, and then defeat it.

HIV becomes deadly only to the uninformed and ignorant people. One might be a carrier without knowing it, which is dangerous because as a carrier, one looks very health and full of life. Late Steve Jobs rightly advised us by saying, "Our time on earth is limited and we don't have to waste it by living someone else's life." He further advised all that "We should not be trapped in a dogma which is living with the results of other peoples' thinking" (Jobs 2005).

Being afraid of what people will say or think when you realize that you are HIV positive does not matter in your life; the noise of other people's opinion will only jeopardize ones inner mind and kill you. Having the courage to look at yourself in the mirror, following your heart and intuition, and promising to be alive for you are what matters. The questions one has to ask are these; what can I do with my life? What can I do to live happily the years assigned to me on earth and what efforts would help me beat HIV? The journey of life is to live in the present with joy; the regrets of yesterday are of no use.

It is not what people would say when they hear about your status that matters, for if HIV is already there in your body, you have to be strong and fight it by controlling and beating it. Once you realize how special, unique and different you are from anyone else, then your path to managing HIV and surviving it will be clear to you. Think about it; if diabetes, high blood pressure, high cholesterol and asthma that are silent killers could be managed and controlled by people, HIV could also be controlled.

In those days, smallpox was a mystery, and deadly disease that killed a lot of adults and children before the scientists and doctors could find out proper cure and inoculations, for the disease. Chickenpox, measles and other contagious diseases followed, but all these are now in the past, and HIV with a question of time, would be a thing of the past as well.

We have to take control of our lives and should not let the opinion of others or the societies control us. As a health-care management person, I have witnessed and seen many people who had lived with HIV for more than thirty years; they fought it, controlled it, and now living happily with their lives. It is not so much the disease that affects the soul and spirit, but rather how we react to it, how we hide it, and how we ignore it.

Chapter Two

People all over the world wondered what life was all about with the stigma of the sickness that put the whole world in early 1980s into a cage of solitude silence. The epidemic of HIV/AIDS was a hush-hush moment for everyone, especially the young, promiscuous, and energetic males and females; the sexually active people in the prime time of life; the innocent men, women, and children who got blood transfusion in the hospital; the new born babies that were infected at birth. The infectious brand-new microbe, according to Dr. Anthony Fauci, "seemed like something for science fiction movie" (Fauci 2011) and the dominant feature of that period in the medical arena was full of confusion and silence.

Dr. Anthony Fauci, head of National Institute of Allergy and Infectious Diseases, further recounted that, "The new disease was a mystery, like a mysterious syndrome" as the medical world had never imagined anything like that. The situation was so bad and sad for the doctor to confess that none of them knew the infectious agent, and the researchers had no precise direction in which to research (Fauci 2011). Dr. Fauci further confirmed that the early years were unquestionably the darkest for the medical scientists and doctors as they were characterized by frustration about how little they could do for their patients, and the whole hospitals all over the world were confused.

Patients were about to die when they were admitted, and their survivals were measured only in months; the only care provided to them was mostly palliative. The patients were frustrated as they looked anxiously at the doctors to cure them or assuredly tell them what was wrong with them, but the doctors had no answers and no clue on what to advise the patients (Engel 2006). The doctors and nurses were also afraid of their own lives and dared to get in contact with the patients. It was a bizarre period throughout the whole world.

The whole of medical profession was left in bewildered with the disease, including the epidemiologists, infectious-disease specialists, and oncologists. Researchers were left pondering on several explanations, but none seemed wholly satisfactory. Whatever the cause was, the doctors clearly observed that the immune system in the infected patient was catastrophically and irreparably breaking down. The central cells in the functioning of the immune system and the T cell lymphocytes were dying off at unsustainable rates (Engel 2006, 8).

The HIV (human Immunodeficiency Virus) was unknown, and transmission was not accompanied by signs or symptoms salient enough to be noticed. By 1980s, HIV had spread to at least five continents, (North America, South America, Europe, Africa, and Australia). The spread was unchecked by awareness or any preventive action; thus, millions of people—young men, women, and children—were infected (Mann 1989). There was a great deal of ignorance about the causes of the condition of HIV/AIDS and how it was spreading.

The breakthrough in the disease research was in 1983 when the Human Immunodeficiency virus, or HIV, was discovered showing that the virus caused AIDS. This discovery helped in developing further tests for the control of the virus, but at that time, according to Dr. Fauci, the desperately ill patients were at the tip of iceberg and about to die (Fauci 2011).

Many people at that time thought the disease was meant for a particular group or sector—the Gay People-but as a global percentage of men and women living with the disease reached a dead heat, it became apparent to all that it had no gender target and had no boundaries. It affected all human beings: homosexuals, hemophiliacs, heroin addicts, heterosexuals, youths, whites, blacks, and children of all races.

The deadly disease HIV/AIDS was first thought to be based only on transmission through sexual contact among the gay men. Hence, medical researchers at that early stage referred to the new disease as gay-related immune deficiency (GRID). Latter, it was proved wrong when the disease started to appear in heterosexual men and women, children, and people who had received blood transfusion, then it became more problem for both the scientists and doctors (Silverstein et al. 2008, 21). Many people with hemophilia had contracted HIV through transfusion of blood and blood products.

People were accidentally exposed to the disease through blood transfusion, and unbelievably, the hemophilia community in America and all over the world-realizing that the virus was also in the blood supply given to them-went public about blood safety. The blood-supply safety then gained national attention over the years through teenager Ryan White, who had hemophilia (Silverstein et al. 2008, 22). This gave a game changer for both the government and the entire communities everywhere in the whole world.

In third world country, especially in Africa-where the blood was not properly screened-many innocent people contracted the diseases right there in the hospitals through blood transfusion, injection needles, syringes, and even in the communities through barbershops, hair salons, and so forth, most of these innocent people were still with the virus moving on, dying early with complications, and none of them were aware on how to check the cause, thus spreading the virus from one generation to another.

Many HIV patients in early 1980s, when their statuses were found out, expressed that the doctors told them they had only a few months to live. They were advised to go home and put their houses in order. They prepared themselves to face death, not knowing how this death came into their body, but many of them are still alive and healthy today after more than thirty years of the epidemic and living well with HIV.

Linda Dahlstrom, health editor for MSNBC.com wrote about Bill Rydwels, who was diagnosed HIV positive in 1985, at age fifty-two. Now Bill had lived to be a senior citizen. He is, at present seventy-nine years old; the doctors now joked with him, that he would live to one hundred years (Dahlstrom 2011). There are so many others like Bill who are still living happily today, beating HIV and putting it down under control. Thanks to the world scientists and medical experts who fought day and night, and arrested the disease to the point that many can now control HIV/AIDS instead of HIV/AIDS controlling human race.

Chapter Three

Jonathan Engel, in describing the virus of HIV that proved to be so troubling to the world, said, "it belonged to a subgroup of the retroviruses called lentiviruses or slow virus that replicates and spread slowly in the host body" (Engel 2006, 60) He compared the virus to a cancer-causing virus that acts fast acting in the body, but he noticed that the HIV replication and spread in the host's body is slowly done. He further equated it with simian immunodeficiency virus, which had its single attack on T4 Lymphocytes cells of human system.

The doctors and scientists noticed that the virus is very dangerous as it has an adaptation that makes it very difficult for treatment and inoculation. HIV virus is very smart, the type that could easily evolve itself out of danger from any antiviral agent that the patient could either ingest or inject (Engel 2006, 63).

Compared to Smallpox, Chickenpox and other viruses, HIV is resistant to vaccine because of in a number of reasons:

1. It is very difficult to vaccinate against.
2. It mutates or copies itself extraordinary rapidly.
3. It attacks only those cells critical to the functioning of the immune system, the T 4cells, also called CD4 proteins. (Engel 2006, 64).

This makes HIV/AIDS closely related to simian immunodeficiency virus (SIV), which attacks immune systems of monkeys.

The discovery of this immune deficiency in a monkey population in Primate Research Center in California, led the researchers to West African Region, where these monkeys naturally dwelled.

Beatrice Hahn, a professor of medicine and microbiology, then confirmed that HIV originated in West African from chimpanzees and was transmitted to the human race. According to her, this animal is a natural habitat for Pan Troglodyte which is the origin of HIV/AIDS.

But some scientists like Worobey and Marx, believed that HIV precursor should be older than thought. They believed Simian Immunodeficiency Virus (SIV) should be at least thirty-two thousand-seventy-five years old; (Worobey 2010), according to genetic analysis found in monkeys in Bioko Island, a former peninsula that separated from mainland Africa after the Ice Age. From their research, they believed simian immunodeficiency virus did not cause AIDS in most of the primates' hosts.

Michael Worobey, who is a professor in the department of ecology at the University of Arizona, and Preston Marx, a virologist, of Tulane University, in that research then raised question about the origin of HIV, which scientists believed evolved from Simian Immunodeficiency Virus (SIV).

These Professors questioned "if humans had been exposed to SIV—infected monkeys for thousands of years, why then did HIV epidemic only began in the 20th century?" They queried that something must have happened to change the relatively benign monkey virus into something potent that could start the epidemic (Worobey & Marx 2010). According to Preston Marx, no one had the knowledge of what that flash point was, but there had to be one.

I strongly agree with Worobey and Marx in their theory, for in most African Countries-especially in West Africa-people kept monkeys or chimpanzees as pets, and they were also used as food in some cultures. There were large markets of "bush meat" obtained from these animals in these cultures for many generations, and there was no history of epidemic HIV/AIDS in those cultures till the twentieth century.

There is doubt in these theories because African Monkeys and Chimpanzees had been there for ages. Why did the epidemic virus of HIV/AID in monkeys' surface this particular period of twentieth century in human race to cause such deadly havoc with pandemic disease? Many people, especially those from African Continent, are still skeptical about the origin of HIV/AIDS emerging from African chimpanzees or monkeys.

There are many questions to be answered. How could we explain the epidemics of HIV in the remote villages of Africa, where there were no traces of monkeys or chimpanzee? And for centuries, people in those cultures had nothing to do with monkeys; still; the epidemics of HIV hit those areas severely in the early 1980s. How can we explain that the great-grandfathers in Africa never had this epidemic all those past centuries?

How can we explain that the slaves that were carried from Africa to many parts of the world never had this virus, or passed the virus to other continents where these slaves were carried to? How can we explain that even the missionaries that went to Africa in those years never contracted nor had any idea about this virus? From history, we learnt that it was malaria from bites of mosquitoes that killed most of the missionaries until they were able to discover medications for combating malaria.

Most doctors, scientists and people in Africa were totally ignorant of the epidemic during the early stage of the disease in 1980s, but now the virus is being ascribed to Mother Africa. The Africans took HIV/AIDS as a white-man-killer disease, spreading fast all over the world. It was first labeled in America homosexual disease in America; in Africa, where homosexual was not known much, it was labeled white man's disease from Overseas. The blacks in African believed the epidemic was not for them but for the Americans and white people and ignored everything about it; that was why it spread like wild fire in Africa.

The origin of HIV/AIDS is still a mystery. No one had proved where this HIV/AIDS emerged from. The mystery and ignorance associated with the virus at that initial stage in 1980's had led to lost of many lives. There were many who died with HIV/AIDS without knowing the cause of their sickness.

In Africa, Doctors and other medical personnel had little or no idea about the disease as in all over the world. This was characterized as a period of confusion and rumors as in other parts of the world. The cause was unclear, and very little was known about the transmission, and public anxiety was high. In Many African nations questions remained unanswered as to the cause of HIV/AIDS and how it was transmitted.

Many myths about the disease in Africa contributed to prejudice surrounding it. Some believed HIV/AIDS could be spread by causal contact with a person who has the disease. Day-to-day contact at work, school, and social settings, like shaking someone's hand hugging-all these were some of the myths believed in transmission of the disease.

Some even believed that using the same toilet, drinking from the same glass, and being nearby when someone with HIV coughs or sneezes helped in spreading the disease. The myth also had it that even mosquito bites, sharing the same silver wares or plates, sharing exercise equipments, or playing sports together with HIV/AIDS disease patient would spread the infection.

Many doctors in Africa informed their patients with HIV, that they had only few weeks to live, and many families ostracized their loved ones to save other members of the family from the death-sentence disease. Some blamed their relations in overseas—especially in America—for carrying the disease to Africa.

HIV infection was also thought to be personal irresponsibility of some people. Religious or moral beliefs led some people to believe that being infected with HIV was as a result of one's immoral fault, which they deserved. There were numerous conceptions with people, thinking that one could contact HIV/AIDS through many things.

Because of all these, people were scared to be tested; some preferred to die rather than having the knowledge that they had HIV. I still remember a closed relative who refused to be tested of HIV, when he was very sick; he preferred to die than be tested of HIV/AIDS. He eventually died, and the death was ascribed to HIV/AIDS.

Another relation was very sick, and got emaciated so much that the doctor, without testing, told him that it was HIV/AIDS. As a married man, he was sincere to the marriage of many years. The wife and the children were not sick. He was so confused and accepted to die with the disease. The family advised him to go to another hospital to be tested; he refused and decided to die instead of another doctor giving him the verdict of death-sentence with HIV that came from nowhere.

The elder brother, who had much influence on him, later convinced him and took him to a more equipped hospital where he was tested; the result was negative. It was found out that he had infection, which was treated, with simple antibiotics, and the man got well immediately; he is still living as of today very-healthy.

Myth remained the single most important barrier and reason too many people were afraid to see doctors to be tested or to seek treatment at that initial stage of the disease. People feared the social disgrace of speaking about the disease or taking precaution. The HIV/AIDS epidemics continued to spread and devastated the cultural society of Africa.

At the time, doctors realized there were needs for education and awareness for the disease in many communities and schools, but the only education passed to people in the 1980s in Africa was the use of condoms, abstinence from sex, and sticking to one's sexual partner. There were no other knowledge that one could contact HIV/AIDS through contaminated blood transfusion, in barber or hair salons, and use of contaminated injection needles, which were the cases for infection for many in Africa. The emphasis was that HIV/AIDS is a death sentence on anyone who had it.

The layman in the village indoctrinated that any one that started losing weight must have HIV/AIDS as the disease draws all the blood in the person till it kills him/her. This increased the stigma of HIV/AIDS, and many people started to eat a lot to gain more weight to show they cannot have HIV/AIDS.

Chapter Four

People that were infected with HIV (Human Immunodeficiency Virus) would slowly develop damaged immune systems which would later become AIDS if not checked. AID (Acquired Immune Deficiency Syndrome) was given to the disease because people acquire the condition rather than inherited it. Although the two abbreviations usually appear together (HIV/AIDS), it is important to understand that HIV is a virus, while AIDS is a syndrome, as a deficiency within the immune system, AIDS is a syndrome with a number of manifestations rather than a single disease (Bartlett and Finkbeiner 2007).

People must understand that once someone is tested positive to HIV, the person would remain a carrier for life. Unlike other antibodies for other infections, once HIV is in the body, it stays in the body. The good news at the present time is that the virus can now be controlled and, in some cases have "functional cure".

It had also been proven that HIV positive people with healthy immune systems who started taking oral antiretroviral medicine soon after becoming infected with CD4 counts between 350 to 550 cells proved 96 percent safer. These people would remain undetectable, thus reducing the risk of transmitting the virus to their HIV-negative partners.

This was published by National Institute of Allergy and Infectious Disease (NIAID) in May 2011. The new study confirmed that early antiretroviral use may be the best medicine for keeping your HIV partner uninfected.

The reality of this disease with two HIV—positive partners, even if they are undetectable, is different. The two partners must protect themselves as the partners with HIV might have different types of HIV virus, and having sex without protection might lead to contracting the other person's type of HIV, which may lead to more complications. The virus from one person might be different from another and may cause more problems in the other partner and may lead to resistance in treatment.

Chapter Five

As mentioned before, the disease is an enemy which could be contracted by any one at any time in life, and the defeat of this enemy disease is to be aware always of safe sex and get tested. Many people, who would not understand this simple message, would surely die. A friend of mine once told me that "ignorance is peaceful" but to me sometimes ignorance is death.

After reading Regan Hofmann's stories on "Alive and Kicking", (Hofmann June 2011, 7), I noticed that many people decided to come out clean of their own stories of HIV. If the beautiful and elegant Regan Hofmann could have HIV/AIDS, this made many realize that HIV/AIDS has a changing phase and it's never meant for a particular person.

A good friend of mine confided in me on how her husband had a blood transfusion when he was sick. He recovered after the transfusion, but no one knew that the blood given to him was contaminated. When she left the country for overseas, the husband was bubbling with good health.

But after a short while, her husband became very sick again; this time, he started to lose weight. The doctors were treating malaria and typhoid fever as usual in African Countries. With her idea of HIV as a health personnel, she then called home, and referred him to a particular doctor, and ordered for HIV test.

The doctor immediately took samples and tested him for HIV and it came out positive. The doctor told my friend the result immediately and sent the husband to a specialist hospital. He was admitted and later released from the hospital and was told what to do. The doctor advised the lady to be tested immediately. Her result came out negative.

The husband was stubborn to accept the fact of the HIV disease and refused to take good treatment. He never wanted to discuss about it; the doctor tried to address the issue, but the man was too stubborn to accept the simple truth. Later in the year, he died. It was the wife who then traced to find out how the husband got the virus. The person who donated the blood to the husband already died of HIV/AIDS.

Because of the stigma associated with HIV in African society, the children and relations were not told. The medication was very expensive then in Africa; at the time, the husband quit going to the doctor and even stopped taking his medication because he never believed the doctors and the HIV thing.

He got complications with pneumonia and died. The doctor advised the lady to be tested again after every six months as the husband must had been full blown AIDS last time they had contact before she left the country. According to the doctor, it may take time for the virus to be detected in some people.

The third time of her test, it came out positive. She refused to accept the result and insisted that she had been tested two times with negative results. In the course of her argument, the doctor advised her to immediately seek for treatment if she wanted to survive the disease. She decided to go to another hospital to be tested, and it came out positive again.

It was then dawn on her that the virus was in her for real. The doctor explained to her that sometimes it takes many months or years incubation period in some people. The first thing that came to her mind was death. She thought that the husband was death; now it would be her turn to die, and the children would be left without parents.

For the past twelve years she had lived with HIV and she is undefeated and has never stopped fighting. She confided in me as a health care worker, I helped her realize that she had to take control of her life. She learnt to work on her mind, body, and attitude from that time on and dedicated her life to fighting HIV.

The doctors also taught her to embrace life positively as there is now a changing phase of HIV/AIDS. She believed that she could save many lives by reaching out to others, especially in Africa, where the stigma is still prominent and many are hiding under the clones of HIV. She then extended to people working in health care with HIV and started to donate to clinics in Africa, for a fight on HIV/AIDS though she remained anonymous.

"There is nothing as damaging to a poisonous secret as its release, when we tell our truth, we own it". (Hofmann 2010). This lady confided only in her children and told them the whole story, and what happened to their father and her. The family supported her in her fight for HIV in Nigeria and backed her up with her donations. The children's understanding and support had bolstered her as much as medical care did.

Stigma remained the most important barrier for treating HIV/AIDS and limited program effectiveness. The related stigma included negative attitudes, abuse, maltreatment, and ostracism. It was one of the reasons why many were afraid to go to the doctor or be tested as it was always associated with moral baggage and personal irresponsibility, especially in Africa.

A married woman in Africa and third world countries, who had been infected by the husband in some areas with male-dominated societies, would always carry the blame and may be killed as they would never accept that the man would be wrong. In those countries, it would be harder for the woman.

The consequences of stigma and maltreatment directed to HIV/AIDS were many; it ranged from being shunned by the families, peers, and wider community. The stigma existed worldwide; it manifest differently in many countries. Even in the United State of America, it was not until fourth of January 2010 all HIV—positive people were restricted from entering the country whether on holidays or visiting on longer-term bases. Thanks to President Barak Obama and his government.

Stigma made it very difficult for people to come in terms with HIV and manage their illness, and worst still, it interfered with the attempt to fight the disease. Many people feared the social disgrace of speaking about HIV, or taking available precautions.

We could fight stigma through education, and enlightenment. Schools, Media houses, and religious leaders should be involved in teaching people to challenge discrimination, stigma, negative discriminatory attitude, and denial they encounter in their society and elsewhere. There should be laws and policies in all societies to encourage freedom of speech and confront the biased social attitudes of all nations in order to be able to fight the stigma that confront HIV/AIDS.

Chapter Six

It is not unusual that being diagnosed with HIV would create a weird emotional conflict. The first impulse to the news of the virus would be anger and range. The patient would be angry to life itself and question why he/she should exist after all. So many adverse feelings would engulf one's personality. The person would be filled with fury for even existing and threaten to commit suicide. Life would be threatened with uncertainty and unpredictability of living with the virus. Many would term it unfair to be singled out by the virus.

The anger of HIV may lead to frustration, depression, fatigue, guilt, and uncertainty of life. Some would be angry in remembering the stigma, rejection, and abandonment that would be associated with HIV. The idea of the virus in one's body may also cause pain. People suffer pain physically and emotionally stemming from the daily humiliations of dependency on drugs for the virus for the rest of one's life and, most importantly, lack of power and moral pain to being forced to make choices. Some people would cry every day because of the anger they felt.

With HIV infection, all these emotions should be natural, justifiable, and appropriate. It is natural to feel this way with any threatening disease. It is also a normal response to having HIV/AIDS, which should affect the brain and ability to suppress emotions. But the most important thing should be to acknowledge the anger that came with the disease and find constructive ways to deal with it. No one wants to die prematurely. According to Steve Jobs, even those who want to go to heaven do not want to die to get there. Yet death is the destination for everyone, for people both positive and negative with HIV/AIDS.

Anger is an emotion, and like any emotion, it could only be held for a short while, for the longer one holds it, the more harm it does to one's body. Suffering may confuse many and cloud their minds; thus, they may not use their reasons clearly. But when we accept these motions, it means we have sentenced ourselves to death and that's exactly what HIV virus wants us to do.

The most important thing we should do in this situation should be to set all these emotions aside. Remember that even the bold seek an escape when they see death approaching. What we should do at this moment would be to prize nothing in life as highly as our well-being and face to fight anything that would prevent us from enjoying life to the fullest. Life is a journey, and on the journey of life, so many bad and good things may happen, but that would never make us to quit enjoying life. We should not be moved by what we see in our journey in life. We have to be in charge of our lives no matter the circumstance, not even the HIV/AIDS.

Josephine, a good friend of mine, who contacted it from one time-relationship, said "why me? I didn't do anything wrong". This girl was a virgin, and the only relationship she had in preparation for marriage got her an HIV infection. She wondered what she did different from what others were doing. This was an unfortunate incident, but there was nothing one could do other than to be courageous and to fight it, for the virus had already entered her body.

When we are faced with the virus, we should find power to confront the situation that led the virus into our lives. Consult the doctor immediately, and attach yourself to a group. The best thing that would ever happen to anyone is belonging to an HIV/AIDS group. This should be formed all over the world. This is where one can discuss and interact with others that have the disease. It is a therapy group that binds people together; they discuss the difficulties they are facing and collectively know how to get on with their lives. The group is like a club and brings a lot of relief to all that belong to it. It helps them to share what ordinarily they could not share with others.

It provides people with HIV with a relaxed and informal place to share their experiences and build new friendships. It further gives HIV couples an opportunity to discuss relational, legal, health, and other issues that concern them.

Chapter Seven

The disease had hit African and many third world countries because most of the hospitals and laboratories were not equipped with the modalities to test HIV/AIDS and to investigate the cause of the virus. The Labs were only equipped with instruments to test many tropical diseases like malaria, typhoid fever, etc.

The doctors were treating acute malaria in many cases when patients with HIV were admitted. It was hard to dictate HIV without adequate test; both the doctors and hospitals were guessing on what was wrong with the patients. The ignorance of the medical people at that period made it to be the most vicious pandemic in the history of Africa. HIV devastated poorer regions, of Sub-Sahara Africa, where the vast majority of HIV positive people lived.

The voices of the concerned individuals and groups in America and other civilized countries sent their governments to vote billions of dollars to research for the disease, but the poor third world nations, especially Africa nations were left to their fate. The poor nations were faced with hunger, deprivation, powerlessness, violation of dignity, social isolation, resilience, gender inequality, etc and were now hit with the deadly pandemic virus.

Poverty is multidimensional and had a psychological dimension that maintained cultural identity and social norms of solidarity, which helped people to continue to believe in their own humanity despite inhuman conditions.

Third world countries and African people lacked basic infrastructures particularly in the rural areas, where transportation, clean water and adequate education were farfetched. Poor health and ill health were dreaded almost everywhere as a source of destitution.

The cost of health care, which poor people could not access, did contribute to HIV/AIDS epidemics and added to a long-term trend in impoverishment. One of the effects of it was that the house-hold of the victim would become poorer. The poor Communities rarely understood the causes of virus, and it became very difficult to assist those affected. Programs for counseling and treatment needed to address the fear of social isolation led individuals to hide the fact of infection.

When charitable organizations and World Health Organizations went to Africa to help with the disease, there was no way to get into the interior parts, because of poor condition of roads. The most frequently cited barriers to accessing adequate health care for people included cost, distance to health-care facilities, and lack of confidence of treatments provided by hospitals and clinics.

Before the United Nations and World Organizations swamped into Africa for HIV/AIDS, the disease controlled the people's lives because of the poor conditions of the people, and it was impossible to get into the interior parts of villages where most HIV people lived. Hence, HIV/AIDS continued to spread rapidly in those areas.

In most African hospitals, several nurses and workers contracted the disease from the patients due to ignorance as many of these nurses were not adequately trained for the job.

Rosaline, a nurse that worked in a private hospital in Africa, in early 1980s during the outbreak of HIV/AIDS when many hospitals never knew what the disease was, contracted the disease. This lady was sick for several years, got married, and had a baby boy. The husband died, and after few years, the lady also died.

Nobody dictated what was wrong with her as she continued working in the hospital. She was tested for everything in the hospital, except HIV/AIDS. The notion was that as a nurse in the hospital, she was prone to contracting the disease. By the time I met her; she had slimmed down so much in weight, and had rashes all over her body.

She could have been alive by now if that awareness were created. She confessed to me that the doctors could not dictate what was wrong with her. She resigned from the hospital to take care of herself in a native way. The family believed that an enemy had inflicted the sickness into her through witchcraft.

She then resorted to herbal treatment and later died. The son also started being sick, from one ailment to another; as a child; he was not tested for HIV/AIDS, as the belief was that HIV could only be contacted through sexual relationships, and as such, children had nothing to do with HIV. When the boy died, the death was also attributed to witchcraft.

I wish I had known what I know now as a trained Health worker; I would have taken that boy to the hospital and insisted on testing for HIV. I am sure that boy would have been alive by now. The death of all the members of that family was one of the things that inspired me to research on HIV/ AIDS. This proved that as a result of condition of poverty and ignorance, people became more vulnerable to HIV/AIDS, as these poor people, with their ignorance, had less access to necessary facilities for prevention and treatment of the virus.

In Africa and many poor third-world-country families, the relationship between HIV and poverty were complex and direct as the capacity to cope with the disease would depend on financial and human endowment of the family. The poorest would be least to cope with the effect of the disease, for even the less poor would find their resources diminishing due to high cost of treatment. An example of this could be seen from the poor nurse whose whole family was wiped out due to ignorance. If she had the means and were properly educated on HIV, she could have gone to a more equipped hospital or clinic and be tested.

The existence of ignorance in many poor nations would be a co-factor in the transmission of HIV. The poor people may understand what they were urged to do for prevention, but that would be impossible if they did not have the urge, the incentive or the resources to adapt to the recommended behavior. For the poor, the programs and policies that were recommended to them would fall on deaf ears. This was observed from the last medical mission that I attended in 2011 in Nigeria on breast cancer awareness with many trained medical teams of a nonprofit organization.

There was this lady whose right breast had been destroyed by breast cancer; she turned down all our pleadings to take her to the hospital for more examination and possible surgery. The Non Profit Organization, I was working with, volunteered to take care of all the financial responsibilities; she still turned down our offer. She stressed that once she was taken to the hospital, her breast would be removed. According to her, "No man would be happy to have a woman without breast". At forty seven years, she had more concern about retaining her breast for a man than fighting for her life.

It was not surprising that the poor, under certain circumstances, would adapt to behaviors which would expose them to HIV infection. This showed that even when the poor understood what they were being urged to do, they lacked the incentive and ignorant to adapt to the recommended behavior.

HIV epidemics would spread due to economic and mind-set poverty, and until this poverty is reduced, there would be little progress either with reducing transmission of the virus or with enhancing the capacity to cope with its social-economic consequences.

During my 2012 medical mission to Nigeria, I met a lady who is now an advocate for fighting the disease in the villages and bringing awareness to many towns about the importance of being tested for HIV and taking medication. A man that tested positive told the lady never to let the wife know about his state. This is one of the problems we have in Africa. The wife tested negative and should know so that both of them would take percussions and live longer, but the man had warned that the wife must never know his status. Such are some difficult situations medical and health-care people face in Africa.

Poor communities rarely understand why they should be inflicted with the virus and how they should assist those affected. Programs for counseling and treatment were needed to address the fear of social isolation, which led many individuals and households to hide the fact that they have the disease.

Many African men rely on informal source of care and simply go without health care. Most of them object to the use of condom for protection as they have negative attitude for it and pass it to the young growing boys; according to them, it reduces the performance.

Chapter Eight

It is very important to know that anyone can be at risk for HIV/AIDS. We now understand that for more than 30 years of the current HIV/AIDS epidemics, no region or country has been spared.

HIV may be found in all the body fluids of an infected person, especially in the blood, semen, and secretions. The virus would be spread when the fluid is transferred from one person to another through open wounds or sores, open cuts, breaks in the skin, unprotected sex, and from mother to her child during birth.

All these can happen through;

- **Sexual contact with an infected person.** Unprotected sex with someone who happened to be either HIV positive or who does not know his/her HIV status would be one of the major ways of transmission of HIV virus. There may be cracks and bleeding of the skin, which would make it fertile for invasion of the HIV virus.

  It should be very important to practice safe sex always because we would not want to expose ourselves to serious illness. If someone is already HIV positive, one could be infected with more dangerous strains of HIV from another person. It could be HIV that was resistant to anti HIV drugs.

  HIV positive people would be at increased risk of getting other diseases like, syphilis, gonorrhea, hepatitis, which are also infectious and deadly; the problem would be that the body may be less able to resist the infection. The use of condom, diaphragm and other protected-sex instruments are highly advised.

- **Sharing needles, syringes, intravenous injections, with an infected person.** If a needle or syringe is reused by another person without being sterilized, the first person's blood may be injected into your blood, causing transfer of the infection if the first person has HIV. The best way to avoid HIV would be to always use a new syringe and needle.

  Most hospitals in Africa and other poor nations had learnt the importance of not sharing needles with patients. But how about the unlicensed quack chemists and untrained nurses who have their own free clinics in these Countries? It is not advisable to get treatments from these road-side chemists and clinics.

- **Mother-to-child transmission**. The placenta joins the pregnant mother to the unborn child. An HIV pregnant woman must let the doctor know immediately so that she would receive treatment to protect the unborn child. If one is pregnant and not sure of her HIV status, please get tested immediately.

  These days, HIV-positive people can have children that are normal, thanks to scientists and doctors. Planning a pregnancy used to be risky for HIV mothers, but today, women with HIV who stay on their treatment and closely monitor their viral load by specialist doctors have a healthy baby. The most important thing is to seek an obstetrician who is also a specialist in HIV. According to Dr. Alice Stek, director of prenatal services at the Maternal, Child, and Adolescent/Adult Center for Infectious Diseases and Virology, at the Los Angeles County-University of Southern California Medical Center, an obstetrician with a strong knowledge of HIV will advise correctly on how to have a healthy HIV-negative baby. Breast feeding is not recommended for HIV-positive mothers

- **Blood transfusion.** This is one of the HIV sources of infection. In the early stages of HIV, the blood banks were not able to tell which of the blood they received that had HIV virus. Now the blood is thoroughly screened for HIV anti bodies before transfusion in most of the countries.

- **Transmission in health care.** Health-care professionals do get infected with HIV in their work place. They could be stuck with needles, syringes, or sharp objects that contained the HIV—infected blood of patients. These days, the health care professionals are very careful in protecting themselves at work. They always use very strong, protective gloves.

The good thing is, the virus had several weaknesses in spreading. It could not survive in the air and it could not penetrate healthy skin or intact epithelial membranes.

Chapter Nine

It is obvious that seven out of ten teens are having sex, and this should not come as a surprise to anyone. Sex education should be very important in our families. As parents and adults, it is very important that we should engage our children to be aware of sexuality; we cannot leave this for the school alone. As long as we deny that our children are having sex at early age, and refuse to teach them comprehensive sex education, our children will remain powerless to defend themselves while gripped by raging hormones. Children contact HIV very early in life because of ignorance from parents, school and society.

The number of children from fourteen to twenty-five years who are infected with HIV is amazing. Globally, younger people in recent times account for more than half of all new HIV cases.

Young people remain at the centre of the HIV/AIDS epidemic in terms of rates of infection, vulnerability, impact, and potential for change. They have grown up in a world changed by HIV/AIDS, but many still lack comprehensive and correct knowledge about how to prevent HIV infection. This situation persisted even though the world had agreed that young people had the human right to education, information, and services that could protect them from harm.

An estimated 11.8 million young people today between fifteen to twenty four years are living with HIV/AIDS, and each day, about 6,000 young people are infected. Many of them at this time are unaware of their status (Piot 2002)

Young people are now at the center of the global HIV/AIDS pandemic as they are the world's greatest hope against this fatal disease.

We as parents and guardians must understand that adolescence is a time of experimentation with drugs, alcohol and sex. Most young ones are crying out to be heard through actions and body movement, but we, the adults, are too busy to attend to them. So many of them get information concerning sex from their friends or from pornographic films and literatures as their parents had never discussed anything about growing up as a man or woman with them.

Parents, extended families, communities, schools, churches etc, are critical in guiding and supporting young people to make safe choices about their health and well being. Consistent positive emotional connections with a caring adult will help young people feel safe and secured, allowing them to develop the resilience needed to manage the challenges of their lives.

Early adolescents from ages 10 to 14 is a time when enduring patterns of healthy behavior can be established, including the onset of sexual activity which can quell the spread of HIV/AIDS (Piot 2002). Establishing healthy patterns of healthy living from start is easier than changing risky behaviors already entrenched.

Educating young people about HIV and teaching them skills in negotiation, conflict resolution, critical thinking, decision making and communication improves their self-confidence and their ability to make informed choices, such as postponing sex until they are matured enough to protect themselves from HIV and other sexually transmitted diseases and unwanted pregnancies.

Chapter Ten

Many people who lost their loved ones and dear friends became interested and come together to urge for solutions to this deadly epidemic disease. Many organizations started to speak out, urging individuals and government to find ways to tackle this deadly virus. Cases of HIV/AIDS were reported worldwide by 1983; in November of that year, World Health Organization Held the first meeting to address the issue.

The World Bank came up with many long-term and short-term specialized and technical support and knowledge for effective care, treatment, and prevention Of HIV/AIDS. It also helped in many ways in alleviation of social and economic consequences for affected communities. The World Bank played leadership role by doing the following:

- Supporting HIV/AIDS strategic plan. This it did by helping countries to develop well-prioritized, evidence-based national AIDS strategies and action plans
- Preventing sexual transmission of HIV, through education
- Strengthening social protection for people affected by HIV

The World Bank helped in many ways in fighting HIV/AIDS and in supporting countries to improve the efficiency, effectiveness, and sustainability of national HIV/AIDS programs. The World Bank worked with stakeholders to improve prevention of HIV by working hand in hand with the sectors of education, transport, energy and infrastructure.

It initiated Global HIV/AIDS Programs (GHAP) for effective management of AIDS programs. The Global HIV/AIDS Program became the central coordinator unit on within the World Bank that supported the effective management of institutional capacity on AIDS.

There were ten cosponsors of UNAIDS, these were International Labor Organization (ILO), Office of the United Nations High Commissioner for Refugee (UNHCR), United Nations Children's Fund (UNICEF), United Nat Nations Development Program (UNDP), United Nations Educational Scientific and Cultural Organization (UNESCO), UNITED Nations Office on Drugs and Crime (UNODC), United Nations Population Fund (UNFPA), World Food Program (WFP), the World Health Organization (WHO), and World Bank. As one of the sponsors, the World Bank helped to share the global response to HIV/AIDS, in partnership with the Nations Government and Non Government Organizations.

The International AIDS society (IAS), was the world's leading independent association of HIV Professionals, with over 14,000 members from more than 190 countries working at the all level of Global response to HIV/AIDS. The members were from all works of life and discipline and included researchers, clinicians, public health and community practitioners on the frontline of the epidemic, and policy and program planners. The International AIDS Society, (IAS) had biennial Conference, where they had interaction on problematic response to the epidemic and ways it could be solved.

The next International AIDS Conference for 2012 was in Washington DC.

The first personality I would love to remember with HIV/AIDS would be Elizabeth Taylor (1932-2011). She was one of the first people to bring National attention to the growing epidemic of the disease. In 1984, Taylor coordinated and hosted the first fund-raiser for AIDS project in Los Angeles. She founded the American Foundation for AIDS Research (AMFAR) in 1985 soon after the death of her friend Rock Hudson in AIDS related illness. In 1986, Taylor testified before the congress for Ryan White bill, and when the legislation was passed in 1993, it helped fund emergency AIDS care for needy areas.

In 1991, she founded the Elizabeth Taylor AIDS Foundation. This was used in focusing on funding AIDS-based service organizations that deliver direct care to people with HIV and provide public education. She raised millions of dollars for this cause, and her organization had given grants to more than 311 HIV related organizations. Taylor vowed to be on a crusade battle against AIDS battle till a cure is found. She died in March 2011, of congestive heart failure at age 79.

President Clinton is another advocator and fighter for HIV/AIDS. He founded the William J. Clinton Foundation, which initiated a global health organization committed to strengthening, and integration of health systems in the developing world. The Foundation was also aimed at expanding care for treatment of HIV/AIDS.

The Clinton Health Access Initiative (CHAI) was to make treatment for HIV/AIDS more affordable and to implement large-scale integrated care, treatment, prevention programs that would help touch many people living with AIDS around the world. These activities included AIDS care in Africa and to more than seventy other countries, including twenty-two governments.

Clinton's organization made it possible for the purchase of AIDS medications and diagnostic equipment at CHAI'S reduced prices. CHAI brought on programs that helped governments in preventing of mother-to-child transmission of HIV/AIDS. In 2007, CHAI partnered with UNITAID, to reduce the price of medication in order to help the middle-income and low-income countries (Clinton Health Access Initiative).

In1999, the World Bank launched the first Global response to HIV/AIDS in Sub Saharan Africa. This was called the Multi Country HIV/AIDS Program for Africa (MAP).

The Inova Juniper is one of the clinics that render help to millions of people with HIV/AIDS. This is one of the clinics that were erected in remembrance of Ryan White, the young thirteen-year old boy that died in 1990 from HIV/AIDS. This clinic is all over United States, providing group meetings, helps, and medical assistance to many people with HIV/AIDs.

Chapter Eleven

This chapter courses the history of more than thirty years war on HIV/ AIDS that changed the course of History in the whole world, as reported by *HIV plus Magazine of July/ August 2012 and HIV Specialist Magazine*, winter 2011. Throughout these years, the war moved from panic and paranoia to the present-day acceptance, tolerance, prevention, and treatment. It was a very severe war, which included the patients themselves, families, Doctors, scientists, politicians, and many reality stars.

- 1981: The first reports of unusual outbreaks of pneumocystis carinii pneumonia (PCP) were reported in United States of America. The Centers for Disease Control (CDC) and Prevention established a task force on the disease and opportunistic infections. This was later identified as AIDS.

- 1982: The Center for Disease Control (CDC) reported 452 cases of the syndrome from 23 States in USA. In that year doctors and researchers gave the disease the name of Acquired Immune Deficiency Syndrome (AIDS).

- 1983: Cases of AIDS were being reported worldwide. In the United States about 3,064, have been infected and 1,292 have died. In May of that year, mayor, Dianne Feinstein declared first week in May as the AIDS Awareness week. In August of that year, activist Michael Callen and many others testified at the congressional hearing on HIV/AIDS. This helped in bringing AIDS alert to the whole world.

- 1984: French and American researchers discovered the virus that they believed to be the cause of HIV/AIDS. This they called

Human Immunodeficiency virus or HIV. In December of that year, a thirteen year old boy from Kokoma, Indiana, Ryan White, was diagnosed with HIV/AIDS, which he contacted through tainted blood, as a hemophiliac. The harassment of White and his family by the community made National news and created more awareness.

- 1985: The first antibodies blood test was licensed by the United States Food and Drug Administration. Ann-Margret and Los Angeles Mayor Tom Bradley participated in the first AIDS Walk. In September of that same year, the American Foundation for AIDS research was formed by Elizabeth Taylor and she promised to put a Hugh sum of money for HIV/AIDS mission. Rock Hudson died of AIDS complications at the age of fifty-nine, in his Beverly Hills Home. Larry Kramer lunched The *Normal Heart* a semiautobiographical play about AIDS epidemic in New York City.

- 1986: In February of that year, President Reagan's administration passed a law rejecting immigrants who tested positive for HIV/AIDS into United States of America. In June, the Federal Government of USA committed one hundred million dollars over five years to evaluate promising AIDS medication.

- 1987: FDA approved the first AIDS drug, AZT. In October, the largest gay-rights march in the USA was held. Activist Cleve Jones unveiled his *NAMES Project Memorial Quilt* to commemorate those lost to AIDS

- 1988: The United States Congress passed an 800 million dollar AIDS research fund. The Center for Disease Control that year helped to distribute the pamphlet *Understanding AIDS* to millions of families in America and all over the world. President H.W. Bush endorsed protections against discrimination for people with HIV/AIDS.

- 1989: Thousands of AIDS demonstrators in New York storm the City Hall to draw attention to AIDS problem in the City and all over America. The *Red Hot organization* organized AIDS Charity, to raise money for HIV/AIDS causes.

- 1990: Congress passed Ryan White Comprehensive AIDS Resources Emergency Act in honor of the brave boy who passed at a tender age, with HIV/AIDS. The Federal Funding would be for a variety of HIV/AIDS related services. In February of that year, artist Keith Haring died of AIDS related complications at age 31. The *Longtime Companion* a very powerful film was released and this focused solely on AIDS. The film educated many people about AIDS.

- 1991: A second anti HIV drug, didanosine, sold under the brand name Videx, was approved by FDA. Also a major research study showed that AZT medication can slow progression to HIV/AIDS systems, but the medication was very expensive.

- 1992: Mary Fisher, HIV positive lady, addressed the Republican National Convention, bringing awareness to the political world the importance of fighting the deadly disease by the whole nation. In December that year, the Bush White House empowered the Food and Drug Administration to fast-track experimental anti HIV/AIDS drugs.

- 1993: *The film Philadelphia,* which starred Tom Hanks, won an Oscar. That same year Tony Kusher's *Angels in America,* Millennium Approaches", earned Tony Award for the Best Play. All these were based on HIV/AIDS epics which brought awareness to many reality stars; this brought many of the stars into war on HIV/AIDS.

- 1994: Pedro Zamora, the 22 years old AIDS activist died of AIDS related complications one day after airing the last episode of *The Real World* and President Clinton publicly thanked him for putting a brave face to HIV/AIDS. In November of that same year, research analysis revealed that AZT medication can cut mother-to-child transmission of HIV by two-thirds.

- 1995: President Clinton in June established Presidential Advisory Council on HIV/AIDS by Executive order. Another antiretroviral drug was approved by FDA called "saquinavir" with brand name "invirase" the first in a new class of drugs for HIV/AIDS called protease inhibitors.

- 1996: International AIDS conference was held at Vancouver, with good news that HIV/AIDS medications so far had transformed the disease from a terminal one into a chronic, manageable disorder like diabetes. The dead sentence on HIV/AIDS was removed to a manageable illness.

- 1997: There was a documented drop in AIDS death. The Center for Disease Development (CDC) officials attributed this to the new drug therapies. In June of that year, Post-exposure prophylaxis or PEP, medication was offered to those who may have been exposed to the virus but have not tested positive yet.

- 1998: The FDA approved the first human trial of AIDS vaccine in United States of America. The joint United Nations AIDS Program announced that HIV/AIDS infection rose 10% worldwide with great increase among women and youth.

- 1999: The CDC reported that there was a great drop of death from AIDS down by 42 percent. The Federal officials confirmed that performance of the new drugs caused people to comfortably fight the disease.

- 2000: The World Health Organization reported that HIV/AIDS stabilized for the first time in Africa. New researches indicated that AIDS could have been around longer than early 1980's.

- 2001: The twentieth Anniversary of HIV/AIDS epidemic-the United Nation devoted a special session to HIV/AIDS and declared it a public health issue. A declaration of Commitment was signed by the whole member countries, which included pledges to reduce HIV/AIDS globally among the young ones by 25% by the year 2010.

- 2002: The FDA approved an HIV/AIDS test can give result in less than 20 minutes. In that same year, the World Health Organization made antiretroviral drugs more accessible to people in poor nations.

- 2003: President W. Bush, in January of that year, approved President's Emergency Plan for HIV/AIDS Relief, (PEPFAR). The main focus of this plan was aimed at fighting HIV/AIDS in Developing Countries. In December of that year, the WHO on the World AIDS Day gave their proposal of "3 by 5" plan, which was that three million people in resource-poor countries would be on antiretroviral drugs by the year 2005.

- 2004: The first PEPFAR fund was disbursed to 14 countries in February that year for about $350 million dollars, approved by the Congress. Designers against HIV/AIDS, in December that year, used pop *cultural components*, to raise media awareness of HIV/AIDS.

- 2005: The WHO plan of "3 by 5" which was started in 2003, was short of its goal, but the treatment saved many lives in many poor countries.

- 2006: Atripla, the first one tablet per day regimen HIV drug, was approved by FDA. This strong, once daily medication was from Bristol-Myers Squibb and Gilead Science and combines three antiretroviral drugs in one.

- 2007: The WHO reported that two million people in low-and middle income-countries are receiving HIV drugs. And it was only 28 percent of those who need the drug. There were still 78 percent of HIV infected people still waiting in those countries.

- 2008: The United Nations HIV/AIDS annual report showed that HIV/AIDS deaths worldwide dropped from 2.2 million in 2005 to 2 million in 2007. In November of 2008, Timothy Brown, "the Berlin Patient" was cured of HIV through a bone marrow transplant given to him to treat his leukemia, by German Doctors. According to Regan Hofmann, "Brown embodies the hopes of scientists and millions living with the virus". (Hofmann 2010).

- 2009: President Barack Obama immediately lifted executive order that had denied U.S aids to international family-planning Organizations, most of them very active in HIV/AIDS prevention. He also promised to lift the United States ban on HIV-positive immigrants and visitors into the United States.

- 2010: State and Federal budget-cut crisis threatened AIDS Drugs Assistance Programs in many places and all over the world. Many drug companies, including Bristol-Myers Squibb, stepped up to provide temporary assistance to these programs.

- 2011: The Secretary General of United Nations, Ban Ki-moon, released a report urging all world leaders to step up and take bold action against the HIV/AIDS epidemics. In March of that year, Elizabeth Taylor died of congestive heart failure at age seventy-nine.

- 2012: Steven Deeks, a researcher and clinical doctor, gave reasons for hope of HIV/AIDS cure. According to him, there are two types of cure, "a functional cure and a sterilizing cure". At present, the functional cure is possible. These are the elite controllers with the absence of therapy and generally remain undetectable for years to decades without therapy. These individuals have powerful HIV—specific T-Cells. The Sterilizing cure would be the absence of HIV/AIDS in the body (Deeks 2012).

- 2013: According to Benjamin Ryan (2013), there is a new understanding of a vaccine for prevention. The just one time HIV vaccine trial, demonstrated moderate effectiveness, which can target the virus. The new insight may lead to a better vaccine down the road. On treatment, the scientists believes that those with undetectable viral load and CD4s, at or above 300, would have 97 percent probability of preventing opportunistic infections, and tests could only be needed only yearly. On the cure, there is a gene therapy on the way, which could create a new way to manipulate the genes of CD4S cells to buffer them against HIV infection. According to Benjamin Ryan, the scientists created the splice in the DNA of the CCRS receptor and added new genes to create multiply layers of resistance to HIV, helping to block the virus entry (Ryan 2013). All these are showing that the scientists are truly very close to the way to cure and defeat of HIV.

Chapter Twelve

According to the report of 2010 Global Snapshot, given by the joint United Nations Program on HIV/AIDS during the World AIDS Day in 2010, the total population living with living with the virus is between 31.1 and 35.8 million, and there were between 2.4 million and 3million in 2008. The positive news was that the number of new infections continued to be down.

North America
Total HIV cases: 1.4 million
New infection: 55,000
AIDS related Deaths: 75,000

Western and Central Europe
Total HIV cases: 850,000
New Infection: 30,000
AIDS related Deaths: 13,000

Caribbean
Total HIV Cases: 240,000
New Infection: 20.000
AIDS Related Deaths: 12,000

Latin American
Total HIV Cases: 2 million
New Infection: 170,000
AIDS Related Deaths: 77,000

East Asia
Total HIV Cases: 850,000
New Infection: 75,000
AIDS Related Deaths: 59,000

Middle East/North Africa
Total HIV Cases: 310,000
New Infection: 35,000
AIDS Related Deaths: 20,000

Eastern Europe/ Central Asia
Total HIV Cases: 1.5 million
New Infection: 110,000
AIDS Related Deaths: 87,000

South and South East Asia
Total HIV Cases: 3.8 million
New Infection: 280,000
AIDS Related Deaths: 270,000

Sub-Sahara Africa
Total HIV Cases: 22.4 Million
New Infection: 1.9 million
AIDS Related Deaths: 1.4 million

Oceania
Total HIV Cases: 59,000
New Infection: 3,900

AIDS Related Deaths: 2,000

(United Nations 2010)

Chapter Thirteen

The Good News of HIV/AIDS

After thirty years of the unknown virus—which later became—HIV/ AIDS many- scientists now believed the end of the Pandemic is possible? The National Institute of Health Allergy and Infectious Diseases had confirmed that "Even in the absence of an effective vaccine to control HIV", it is now certain that, "treatment of HIV/AIDS is a prevention that would ultimately end the HIV/AIDS pandemic" (Hoffman 2011).

These scientists had given us a firm impression that treating people who are living with HIV would stop the spread of disease and make the world a better place for all of us.

The prevention interventions of HIV would solely rely on antiretroviral drugs (ARV), which would include prevention of mother-to-child transmission (PMTCT), postexposure prophylaxis (PEP), and highly active antiretroviral therapy (HAART) all had been tested and proved. There are promising results in clinical trials coming from these researches.

After years of battle with the endemic, it is believed that if a drug can lower the viral load of HIV/AIDS, the same drug can help to abort HIV infection before it takes root in the body. The researchers and scientists believed there are many breakthroughs which were merely wishes, and "slowly these wishes are becoming realities and have been translated into standard of cure" (Kalibala and Littlefield 2010).

With these antiretroviral based Microbicides researchers transformed the wishes in 2010 and received awaited proof of concept with positive result. The study was focused on safety and the potential impact of a daily preventive drug on HIV/AID's risk behaviors, which provided more useful information on the relationship among adherence, perception of treatment, and individual risk behavior, as well as feasibility of PEP (Postexposure Prophylaxis).

There would be many setbacks and implications, which may include the cost, provision of ARV and PEP supply that may affect the effectiveness of the program. As both ARV—based microbicides and PEP would be through prescription, it may be difficult for HIV/AIDS negative people to get prescription as these could not be offered through over the counter as condom.

The success of this ARV—based microbicides would depend on community education, accessibility, and confidential counseling services. ARV-based Microbicides is still as part of a package of prevention intervention, and then PEP will need regular testing and partner disclosure.

The study of recent safety involving ARV-based microbicides and PEP has given us hope and anticipation into the field of HIV/AIDS prevention intervention. It is important to know that treating people living with HIV/AIDS will go a long way to ending the spread of HIV/AIDS. Though there may be some programmatic implications as the scientists move forward in the operations research for efficient and effective delivery of this, the physicians and clinical scientists, would address these problems just like they did to other virus of the past decades.

Chapter Fourteen

There is now a game—changing breakthrough in our understanding of both how HIV/AIDS works and the methods we can use to best combat the virus. As there is now treatment that works as prevention in people living with HIV/AIDS as well as those who are not, this shows that with time, HIV/AIDS would eventually be dead as smallpox, chickenpox, polio, and other virus that once terrorized humans all over the world.

The most important thing is that HIV has been defeated; the long-waged battle between the treatment and prevention is over. The fact that antiretroviral treatment is double prevention of HIV for infected people has given us the hope that even in the absence of an effective vaccine, the end of the pandemic is near.

Most importantly, the idea of functional and sterilizing cure is a big hope for cure. It is also recorded that about fourteen people with HIV who were treated with antiretroviral therapy early in their infection have now achieved "viral controller" status without remaining on medication for years. Findings like these have show "functional cure", for though the virus still lives in their bodies, it does little or no harm.

Most importantly, I had witnessed and interviewed a lady who confessed during HIV group, that for ten years she had been off all antiretroviral medications because her body could not tolerate any medication and she had been fine, with no sickness all the years. This is true evidence that "functional cure" is real and the cure for HIV is very near.

References

1. Bartlett, J. G., & Finkbeiner, A., (2007), The Guide To Living With HIV Infection, John Hopkins University Press Health Book, Sixth Edition, Baltimore, MD

2. Connolly, S. (2003), Just The Facts AIDS, Reed Educational & Professional Publishing, Chicago, Illinois

3. Deeks, S., (2012), Towards an HIV Cure, from POZ.com, December, p.14 and 15

4. Dahlstrom, L., (2011), Aging with AIDS: More are living Longer, Living with loss, from, http://www.msnbc.msn.com/ClearPrintProxy.aspx?unique=1307551681216, printed on June 8, 2011

5. Dahlstrom, L., (2011), Aging with AIDs, http://linda-dahlstrom.newavine.com/

6. Engel, J. (2006), The Epidemic, A Global History of AIDS, Smithsonian Books, In Association with, Harpper Collins Publishers, NY, NY

7. Fauci, A., S., (2011), After 30 years of HIV/AIDS, real progress and much left to do, Published May 27, from http://www.washingtonpost.com/opinions/after/30-years-ofhivaids-real-progress-and-much, Reprinted on June 8, 2011

8. Garcia, M., (2011), 40 Weeks to a Healthy Baby, HIV-positive and want to have a baby? Proceed with caution and care, from www.hivplusmag.com/29 March/April

9. Gifford, A., Lorig, K., Laurent, D., & Gonzalez, V., (2005), Living Well With HIV And AIDS, Bull Publishing Company Boulder, Colorado

10. Hahn, B., (2011), The Origin of HIV/AIDs, from http://uhavax.hartfort.edu/bugl/rise.htm, printed September 222022

11. Hofmann, R., (2011), Retiring the Ribbon, poz.com/October November 2011, Twitter @reganhofmannandcheckoutblogs.poz/regan

12. HIV Plus Magazines, www.hivplusmag.com (2010-2012), Merck Sharp & Dohme Corporation, a Subsidiary of Merck & Co., Inc

13. HIV Specialist Magazine, www.aahivm.org (2011), Winter Volume 3, Number 1, by the American Academy of HIV Medicine

14. Kalibala, S., and Littlefield, S., (2010), Treatment Issues, The Role of ARVs in HIV Prevention: Microbicides and PrER, POZ Magazine, poz.com, p. 25-26

15. Mann, J., (1989), AIDS: A Worldwide Pandemic, Vol. 2, Edited by Gottlieb, M. John & Son

16. Piot, P., (2002), Executive Director UNAIDS, Young people and HIV/AIDS Opportunities in Crises, produced by UNICEF Editorial and Publications Sections Division of Communication

17. POZ Magazines, (2010-2013), Merck & Sharp Dohme, Corporation, a Subsidiary of Merck & Co., Inc

18. http://web.worldbank.org/WBSITE/EXTERNAL/COUNTRIS/AFRICAEXT/EXTAFR

19. Ryan, B., (2013), Research Notes: Prevention, Treatment, Cure, concern, POZ Magazine, poz.com, p. 33

20. Silverstein, A., Silverstein, V., & Nunn, S., The AIDS Updates, (2008), Enslows Publishers, Inc.,

21. Support Groups: Places of Healing, HIV/AIDS Focus paper #23, of March 1994, from http://gbgmumc.org/health/hivfocus023.cfm printed on Sept. 30,

22. The Thirty Years War, (2011), from www.hivmag.com, July/August, p.25-29

23. Worobey, M., and Marx, P., (2010), Island Biogeography reveals the deep history of SIV, Science New York, NY, 329(5998)

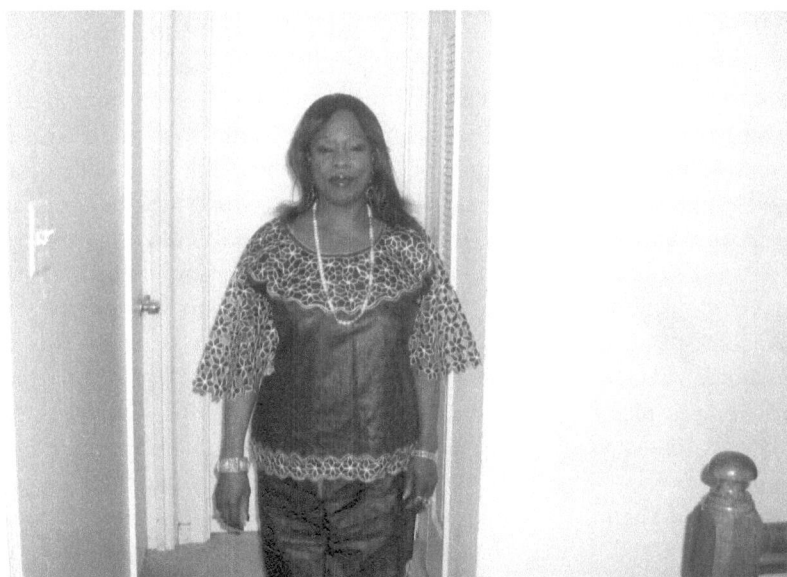

Catherine Ifeoma Elebo (nee Ike), was born and raised in Anambra State of Nigeria. She is the second child in the family of four children and the only girl of the parents.

In 1977 she migrated to the USA with her husband Edwin Elebo and achieved her undergraduate degree in Political Science in 1980, with honors (Magna Cum Laude), graduated with Masters Degree in Education (M.ED), in 1981, all from Texas Southern University, Houston Texas. In 2008, she completed another Master degree in Business Administration (MBA), from Colorado Technical University, in Health Care Administration, and currently a Doctorate Degree student, from North Central University, Arizona, in Health Care Management.

In 1982, Catherine returned with her husband to her home country where she taught at Nnamdi Azikiwe University, a Federal University in Nigeria. She held high profile political and government positions that include; served in the State House of Assembly as the assistant to the clerk of the House, and in the Anambra State Government House, as the Political Advisor, and Chief of Protocol to the Military Governor's wife's office. She was also one of the Chief Supervising Principals in Anambra State Education Commission for many years.

Catherine Ifeoma Elebo had published and co-authored many books for the university which includes; Social Science for Tertiary institutions, Introduction to Philosophy and Logic, Humanities, Nigerian Socio Political Development; Issues and Problems, Issues in Nigerian Development, Social Science and Humanities for Nigerian University.

As a humanitarian, Catherine helped her State in Nigeria to fight for gender equality and human rights for all. She fought for positive changes and elimination of many harmful practices that lead to marginalization of women in Nigerian culture and helped in organizing better life for rural women, family support programs, and women affairs ministry for women self reliance. She is a life member of African women Scholars, and women in Africa and the African Diaspora (WAAD): Health & Human Rights.

In 1998, Catherine relocated back to USA and dedicated herself as a community worker who had devoted extensively to less privileged in Washington DC Metropolitan area USA, through African Humanitarian Council, as the chairperson of the organization. She had volunteered to work in many medical missions in the villages of Africa, especially in Nigeria for so many years, giving lectures and talks on health awareness issues. She helped in Initiating micro credit finance to less privileged women in Anambra State of Nigeria, through Anambra State Association in Americas (ASA USA). She is a board member of Nissi Helps Foundation, a Non-Government, and non-profit Organization (NGO), that is born out of desire to help the less privileged, widows, orphans, and youth empowerment in Africa. The headquarters is at Awka, Anambra State Nigeria. She is also a board member of Oba board of Directors, Oba development foundations, USA, a philanthropic and non-profit organization for the less privileged children in Oba town, in Anambra State Nigeria, and in the Diaspora.

Catherine has received a chieftaincy title by merit, a rare recognition for women in Igbo culture, by the president of the traditional leaders in Anambra State of Nigeria, His Royal Highness, Igwe Peter Chukwuma Ezenwa, for her contributions to gender ideals of equality in human rights, multiculturalism, and resistance to all forms of cultural domination that prevents feminist proactive in our society.

Catherine was the President and CEO of Kkache Health Care Enterprises, a company that delivers efficient home health services for the elderly and disabled in Northern Virginia and Washington DC Metropolitan areas in USA.

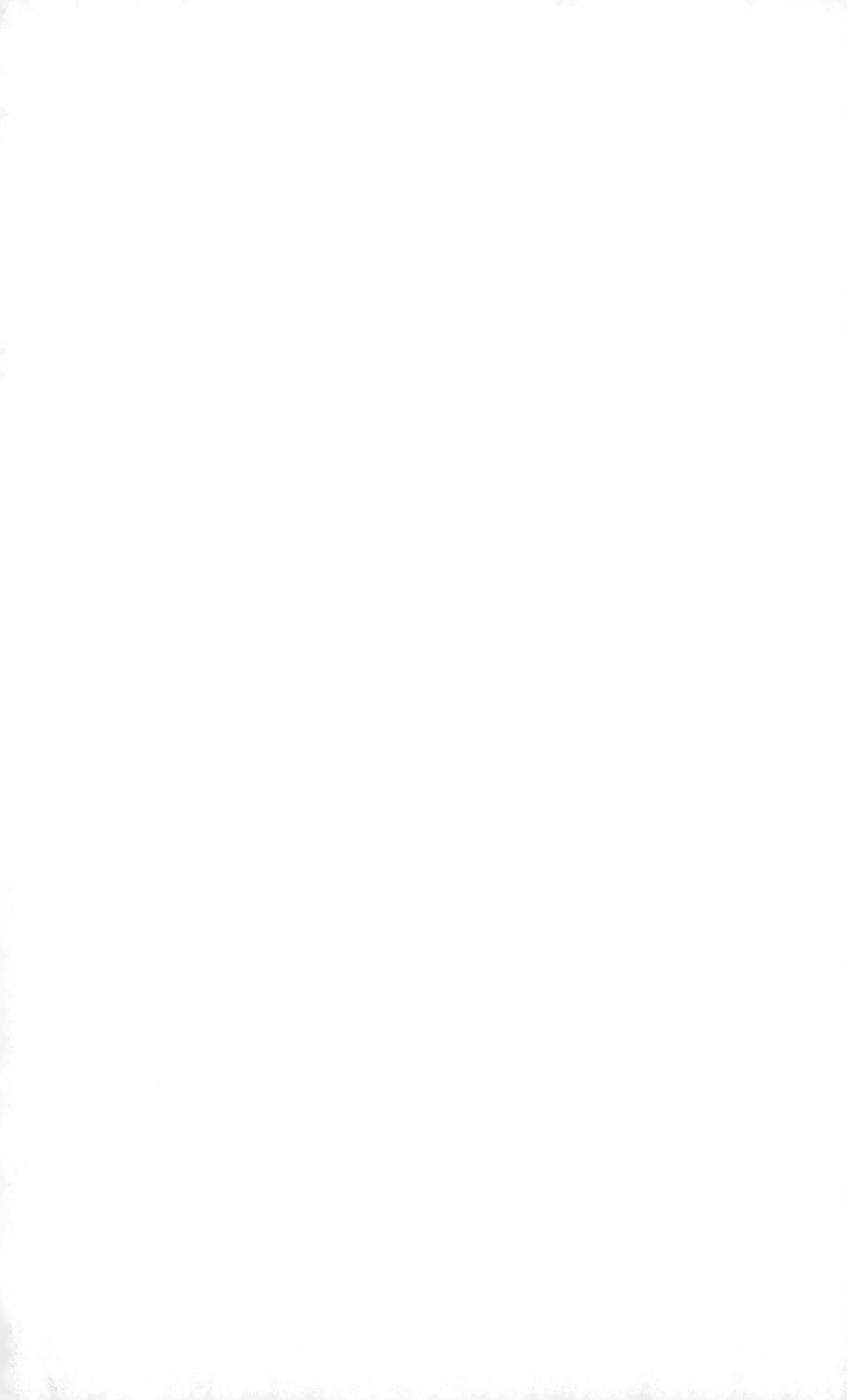

www.ingramcontent.com/pod-product-compliance
Lightning Source LLC
Chambersburg PA
CBHW021935170526
45157CB00005B/2319